YOUR KNOWLEDGE HAS VALUE

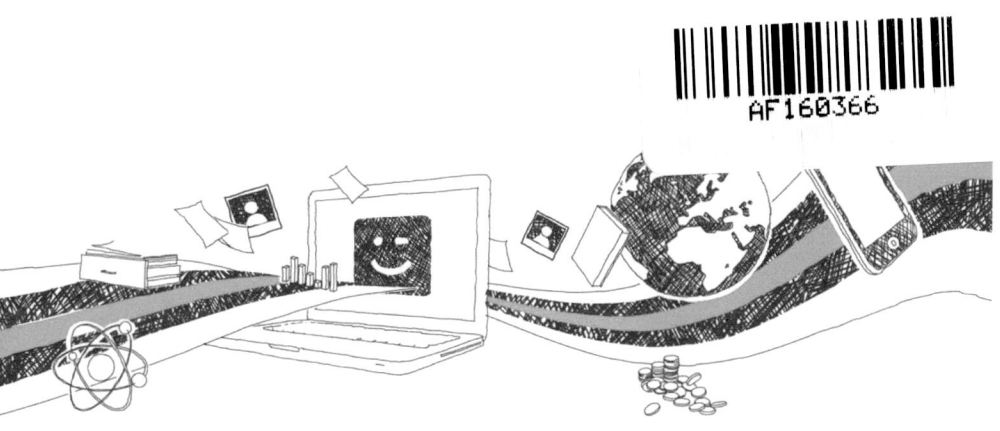

- We will publish your bachelor's and master's thesis, essays and papers

- Your own eBook and book - sold worldwide in all relevant shops

- Earn money with each sale

Upload your text at www.GRIN.com
and publish for free

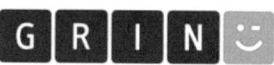

Bibliographic information published by the German National Library:

The German National Library lists this publication in the National Bibliography; detailed bibliographic data are available on the Internet at http://dnb.dnb.de .

This book is copyright material and must not be copied, reproduced, transferred, distributed, leased, licensed or publicly performed or used in any way except as specifically permitted in writing by the publishers, as allowed under the terms and conditions under which it was purchased or as strictly permitted by applicable copyright law. Any unauthorized distribution or use of this text may be a direct infringement of the author s and publisher s rights and those responsible may be liable in law accordingly.

Imprint:

Copyright © 2017 GRIN Verlag
Print and binding: Books on Demand GmbH, Norderstedt Germany
ISBN: 9783668626416

This book at GRIN:

https://www.grin.com/document/384370

Patrick Kimuyu

Cancer Research. The Biology of Gastric Cancer

GRIN Verlag

GRIN - Your knowledge has value

Since its foundation in 1998, GRIN has specialized in publishing academic texts by students, college teachers and other academics as e-book and printed book. The website www.grin.com is an ideal platform for presenting term papers, final papers, scientific essays, dissertations and specialist books.

Visit us on the internet:

http://www.grin.com/

http://www.facebook.com/grincom

http://www.twitter.com/grin_com

Cancer Research: The Biology of Gastric Cancer

Name: Patrick Kimuyu

Inhaltsverzeichnis

Introduction 3

Biological Changes during Onset and Progression of Gastric Cancer 3

Distinctive Characteristics of Cancer Cells 5

Effect of Gastric Cancer in the Body 5

Therapies for Gastric Cancer.. 6

Lifestyle Changes in Gastric Cancer Prevention and Treatment............................... 7

Relationship between Gastric Cancer and other Cancers 7

References 8

Introduction

From a pathological perspective, cancers occur due to the failure of the immune system. It is evident that the immune system plays key roles in preventing cancer through regulating cell population in the body (Dicken et al., 2005). Ordinarily, the body's immune system is usually involved in some cellular processes, especially in the cell cycle in which it destroys old or defective cells through programmed cell death, a process commonly known as apoptosis. In the context of cancer, this process is usually impaired, thus damaged or defective cells are not destroyed by the immune system. In addition, the impairment of the immune system's activity affects cellular homeostasis processes including irregular cell division. These factors are responsible for tumor growth and progression of cancer. Gastric cancer affects the digestive system, primarily the stomach. Anatomically, the stomach occupies the region from the esophageal junction to the duodenum (Cabebe, 2015). Therefore, aim of this research is to carry out a comprehensive review of gastric cancer, also known as stomach cancer.

Biological Changes during Onset and Progression of Gastric Cancer

In gastric cancer, biological cellular changes occur due epigenetic modification of genes involved in maintaining the integrity of cells. These genetic alterations are responsible for changes in cell structure and behavior. One of the key changes caused by mutations of the key genes in gastric cells is changes in gene expression. It is apparent that gene alterations influence the amount of cellular proteins produced by gastric cells. Second, genetic alterations result into the production of defective or abnormal protein products that do not play their cellular biological roles or alter the function of other proteins in the cell. In gastric cancer, there are several molecules which structural alterations. Some of these molecules include the cell cycle regulator (cyclin E) the apoptosis inhibitor (bcl-2), multifunction protein (beta-Catenin), epidermal growth factor, cell adhesion protein (E-cadherin), and plasmolagen activator. On the other hand, some of these molecules exhibit alterations in gene expression. For instance, gastric cancer cells exhibit gene amplification that is responsible for overexpression of K-sam and c-erbB2 proteins which act as growth factor receptors (Becker, Keller & Hoefler, 2000).

Some of the key genes whose epigenetic modifications lead to the development of gastric cancer are CDH1 gene, TP53 gene and APC gene. CDH1 regulates the expression E-cadherin of epithelial cadherin which is involved in cell-cell adhesion, cell movement and cell signaling. Therefore, gene alterations on CDH1 impair the development of organized tissues due to changes in cytoskeletal structures. These alterations have also been found to lead to the development of gastric cancer because it acts as a tumor suppressor gene. On the other hand, mutations on TP53 gene lead to the production of abnormal p53 protein which plays key roles in immune system surveillance. Clinical investigations reveal that TP53 protein is either lost or damaged in 80 percent of gastric cancers. Finally, alterations in APC gene impairs cell signaling within gastric cells (Zheng, Wang, Ajani & Xie, 2004).

At the organ level, gastric cancer causes several biological changes. Clinical studies indicate that noncohesive tumor cells infiltrate the stomach wall. This process leads to glandular formation that does not function as normal gastric glands. In addition, lesions occur on the gastric wall in which diffuse tumors cause inflammation and desmoplasia (Dicken, Bigam, Cass, Mackey, Joy & Hamilton, 2005). Moreover, notch signaling in gastric tumorigenesis appears specific for gastric cancer (Kim & Shivdasani, 2011).

Distinctive Characteristics of Cancer Cells

In practice, the appearance of tissues and organs is determined by the types and arrangement of cells that constitute specific tissues or organs. Cancer is usually identified on the basis of the normal appearance of tissues. Therefore, the distinction between characteristics of cancer cells and normal cells is paramount in pathological investigations of cancer. From a pathological perspective, a comprehensive distinction can be guided by three core features; shape and size of the cells, nucleus appearance and the arrangement of cells in tissues. Ordinarily, normal cells exhibit consistency in the size and shape. In contrast, cancer cells lack consistency, they are either smaller or larger than normal cells, and their shapes are distorted due to cytoskeletal changes. Second, cancer cells have larger and darker nucleus compared to normal cells. Finally the arrangement of normal cells possesses characteristics which are specific to a certain tissue or organ. For instance, gastric cells form glands that produce mucus to protect the gastric wall, digestive enzymes and gastric acid that aid digestion. In contrast, gastric cancer cells form distorted glands. Another significant difference between normal gastric cells and gastric cancer cells is that, normal cells are localized implying that they stay within the gastric walls. This localization is absent in gastric cancer cells because they spread to other surrounding tissues during the progression of the disease, a phenomenon known as metastasis (Duffy, McGowan & Gallagher, 2008).

Effect of Gastric Cancer in the Body

The pathophysiology of gastric cancer explains how the disease affects the body as it progresses. The enlargement of tumors disrupts stomach distension and bowel obstruction. In some cases of ulcerative tumors, bleeding occurs, and this is manifested as melena, gastrointestinal hemorrhage or hematemesis. In advanced gastric cancer, ascites and hepatomegaly occur, ad this implies the impairment of vital homeostasis processes. For instance, hepatomegaly leads to the disruption of the production and release of bile salts. On the other hand, stagnation of lymphatic fluid in tissues causes edema in lower extremities (Dicken et al., 2005). It is also reported that the secretion of gastric enzymes and acid becomes upset as gastric cancer progresses. In most cases, gastric cancer is associated with excessive release of gastric acid due to impaired regulation.

Therapies for Gastric Cancer

Treatment and management of gastric cancer are aimed at preventing the spread of the cancer, especially during its early stages of development and relieving the symptoms associated with the pathophysiology of the disease including control of normal homeostasis in the body. Currently, there are several therapies for the treatment of gastric cancer. Some of the main therapies include surgery, radiation and chemotherapy. Surgery involves the removal of tumors, in order to prevent the progression of gastric cancer. It also removes obstructive tumors in the stomach to enhance distension of the stomach and flow of gastrointestinal contents. On the other hand, radiotherapy destroys tumor cells and prevents it from spreading to other vital organs. Finally, chemotherapy involves the use of therapeutic agents to address the physiological aspects of the disease. For instance, some drugs inhibit tumor cell growth leading to the shrinking of tumors, whereas others treat the symptoms of the disease including inflammation and nausea. Some of the most common regimens involve a combination of cisplastin, leucovorin, epirubicin, and etoposide with ECF infusion. Others include oxaliplatin, irinotecan and taxanes (Dicken et al., 2005).

Lifestyle Changes in Gastric Cancer Prevention and Treatment

Gastric cancer is known to be associated with some lifestyle choices. Therefore, lifestyle changes play significant roles in the prevention and treatment of the disease. Some of the lifestyle choices that increase the risk of gastric cancer are tobacco use, obesity, diets low in vegetables and fruits, and high in pickled and salted foods. Alcohol consumption is also a risk factor. In addition, environmental factors such as exposure to fumes and dust are known to increase the risk of gastric cancer.

My approach to these modifiable cancer factors include weight management and physical exercise to prevent obesity, adoption of a prudent diet with plenty of fruits and vegetables, in order to strengthen the body's immunity against H. pylori infection and avoidance of tobacco smoking and alcohol moderation.

Relationship between Gastric Cancer and other Cancers

It is apparent that some biological changes in gastric cancer are similar those of other cancers. For instance, cancers that are caused by epigenetic modifications of CDH1 gene and APC gene show cellular and molecular similarities. These cancers include prostate cancer and lobular breast carcinoma that are caused by mutations in CDH1 gene. On the other hand, mutations in APC gene also cause colorectal cancer (Zheng, Wang, Ajani & Xie, 2004).

Conclusion

Conclusively, gastric cancer affects the stomach. It occurs primarily due gene mutations in gastric cells which lead to the growth of tumors. Tumor cells assume different morphological characteristics during the disease's progression. Its effects on the body are characterized by hematemesis, ascites and hepatomegaly, especially during advanced stages. This cancer can be treated through therapeutic approaches; whereas lifestyle changes underpin its prevention.

References

Becker, k., Keller, G., & Hoefler, H. (2000). The use of molecular biology in diagnosis and prognosis of gastric cancer. *Surg Oncol.*, 9(1), 5-11.

Cabebe, E. (2015). *Gastric cancer.* Retrieved from http://emedicine.medscape.com/article/278744-overview#showall

Dicken, B., Bigam, D., Cass, C., Mackey, J., Joy, A., & Hamilton, S. (2005). Gastric adenocarcinoma. *Ann Surg.*, 241(1), 27–39. doi: 10.1097/01.sla.0000149300.28588.23

Duffy, M., McGowan, P., & Gallagher, W. (2008). Cancer invasion and metastasis: changing views. *J Pathol.*, 214, 283-93.

Kim, T., & Shivdasani, R. (2011). Notch signaling in stomach epithelial stem cell homeostasis. *The Journal of Experimental Medicine*, 208(4), 677-688. doi: 10.1084/jem.20101737

Zheng, L., Wang, L., Ajani, J., & Xie, K. (2004). Molecular basis of gastric cancer development and progression. *Gastric Cancer*, 7(2), 61-77.

YOUR KNOWLEDGE HAS VALUE

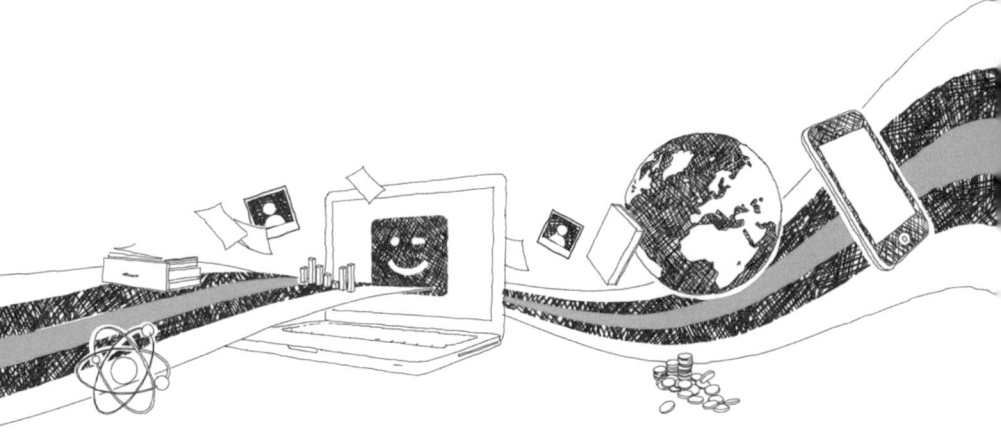

- We will publish your bachelor's and
  master's thesis, essays and papers

- Your own eBook and book -
  sold worldwide in all relevant shops

- Earn money with each sale

Upload your text at www.GRIN.com
and publish for free

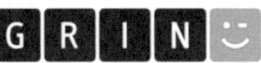